Muckin' About
on the Mat

After investigation, believe that which you have tested and works for you

By the Elephant's Child,
AKA Bob Insley

Thank you Zoe
For steadying the sometimes
crazy ship

Bob Insley

Muckin' About on the Mat
With the standing postures

Copyright © 2021 Bob Insley

ISBN:
978-1-80227-183-6 (Paperback)
978-1-80227-184-3 (eBook)

Contents

Thank you

To every tutor I have ever worked with; some taught me to listen, some to obey, and the special ones taught me to think for myself.

For every person who ever came to classes with myself and Be and returned for more of my stories and horrendous jokes, mostly the same ones told over and over again. Bless you all.

To Antonia Boyle, who kind of started it off.

To Zoe Knott, who it has been my pleasure to work with for over twenty years, and who has listened patiently to my sometimes crazy ideas, and who has added most of the punctuation to my ramblings that have ended up as this book.

To David Kirk, who really was the driving force that encouraged me to start the damn thing in the first place, and has made the final draft look so much better.

To Bex Papa Adams, for demonstrating that my six weeks of struggling with the crooked man can be mastered in about ten minutes.

Especially to Be, for her constructive honesty and patience, for, as I am sure you will know, I can go on a bit.

Thanks to you all for being on my yoga journey with me, but most of all for being my friends.

Bob

Foreword

This book is not an attempt to explain how yoga asana should be done, through some new inspired approach.

It is not particularly comprehensive in the number of asana that it considers, for it only looks at standing postures. It is, in fact, quite limited in this area.

Further, it will not make you super strong, nor super flexible, nor lead you to enlightenment.

What it will encourage you to do is to question, internally and externally, every instruction that a tutor may give you; for it is important to remember that the tutor knows nothing about how your particular mind and body works, but can only give generalisations relating to their own personal experience.

This approach, if you allow it, will enable you to begin to listen to the questions that asana themselves ask and find your own route around and through each posture and the activity that the shape proposes.

To this end, we will look at some asana in detail and reflect on both the instructions, their rationale and reasoning for doing them in a particular way. We will look at other asana, where observations and enquiry may be fleeting.

If you get into the habit of enquiry, then each asana and each action within that asana, will pose the same question – WHY? This alleviates the need for me to write about dozens of asanas because the reality of enquiry will be to ask WHY? no matter the practice. All I will include will be a questioning process and the journey along the path that my thoughts and ideas have led me down.

Let us consider one of the great enquirers and consider the advice that is given. The Kalama Sutra, attributed to the Buddha, sets out a series of suggestions that will enable each individual to find their own way, and in my view, puts the tutor in their rightful place. QUESTIONED!

Here is what the Sutra suggests:

> *Do not believe in the strength of traditions, even if they have been*
> *held in honour for many generations and in many places.*
> *Do not believe anything because many people speak of it.*
> *Do not believe in the strength of sagas of old times.*
> *Do not believe that which you yourself imagined, thinking a god*
> *has inspired you.*
> *Believe nothing which depends only on the authority of your*
> *masters or priests.*
> *After investigation, believe that which you yourself have tested*
> *and found reasonable, and is for your good and that of others.* (1)

Those 92 words encapsulate everything this book encourages.

So really, I guess, I should end the book here and leave you to it. However, what I shall attempt to do instead will be to relate my experiences, thoughts, ideas and suggestions to allow you to find your own way.

As already said, this is not a book of instructions about how to do yoga asana. It is a book that encourages enquiry, giving suggestions and encouragement for each individual to question the nature of the practices themselves. I will, at times, describe an approach that I take. That is all it is; a route that I have found useful for me.

It is not THE right way, but A way that you may consider with all the others. What I will do is explain WHY I have found it useful for me, and give a rationale. The rest is up to you.

First, consider what our individual requirements might be from an asana. Secondly, enquire what the asana or the tutor's instruction asks of us as an individual. We can then perhaps begin to find a middle way between the question 'what do I want from the asana', the instructions and our ability to carry them out.

Tutors have the privilege of offering a journey to other individuals. Tutors should accept and begin to understand their own abilities and restrictions. This enquiring approach may give a window through which we can look and appreciate the ability of other individuals, and adjust our teaching accordingly.

The artist and teacher, Gustave Moreau, often referred to as an "awakener of others", puts it brilliantly when considering his role as a teacher:

"I am a bridge over which some of you may travel" (2)

Now that is a true tutor; humble.

I am reminded of Rudyard Kipling's *Just So* animal stories. (3). One in particular – *The Elephant's Child*. Elephant's Child was a child of insatiable curiosity and asked questions constantly. The questions drove the parents and all other jungle animals mad, for he asked all of them regularly. Because of his insatiable curiosity, Elephant's Child was often beaten for its trouble.

One day, Elephant's Child asked, *"What does Crocodile have for dinner?"* Well, he was sorely beaten by all he asked until he came to the banks of a river where he met Python, the biggest snake in the world.

Elephant's Child asked Python, *"What does Crocodile have for dinner?"* Elephant's Child expected a beating. Instead, Python said, *"Ask him, for Crocodile is in the river just over there."*

Elephant's Child went to the river and called to Crocodile, *"Crocodile, what do you have for dinner?"*

Crocodile replied, *"Well, today, I think I will have Elephant's Child,"* and with this, he grabbed Elephant's Child by the nose.

Now, it is important to remember that at this time, Elephants had massive bulging noses spread across their faces. It was this that Crocodile grabbed, and began to drag Elephant's Child into the water. Well, Python felt bad about this, as it was Python that had encouraged Elephant's Child to ask. So, Python wrapped one end of himself around a rock and the other end around Elephant's Child's leg. Crocodile pulled. Elephant's Child pulled and Python pulled, and what happened was that Elephant's Child's big flat nose became longer and longer until it reached the floor.

Crocodile tired of the tug-o'-war and let go. Elephant's Child thanked Python and journeyed home. On the way home, every animal asked him where he got his long nose from, and what was he going to do with it? Elephant's Child said, "Well, it's much better for me to beat you with, as you beat me for asking questions."

The moral of the story is that if you ask enough questions, you end up with something better than you started with.

So, enquire away, and be one with Elephant's Child on your yoga journey.

Before we get into the asana, it would be great to consider an aspect that relates to every asana that we practise, and consider it every time as we begin any activity.

"What restricts us most in any asana?"

Physically: It may be that parts of the body will limit movement – the feet in contact with the floor, for example. For once they are in a fixed position, this needs to be accepted unless these points of contact can be altered.

Mentally: It may be our perception of what the asana is and our belief that it is necessary to get the body to fit itself into a preconceived mould.

CHAPTER 1

Tadasana

Tall or Mountain posture

Let us start with Tadasana, Samasthiti, mountain or tall posture or whatever other name has been used to describe it. Let's not get too hung up on the wording; after all, it's about standing upright, aligned and at ease. Initially, it will be how we place the feet that will set the scene for the rest of the journey.

With that in mind, let's consider some of the instructions that I have received about feet position:

1. *Outer borders of the feet in line.*
2. *Inner borders of the feet in line.*
3. *Bring the ankle bones together*
4. *Big toe joints touching.*
5. *Lift the inner arches.*

Let's have a look at some of these instructions by taking a look down at our own feet.

1. *Outer borders of the feet in line.*

Well, looking at my feet, if I carry out this instruction, I end up pigeon-toed, and my knees rotate inwards. I cannot achieve 2 or 3, as it's a physical impossibility in this position. The inner arch just naturally lifts in this position, and my big toes touch, so success in three of them, but abject failure in the other two.

What is it like for you?

Now apply this to the other suggestions, and any others you may have been given. Away you go:

2. *Inner borders of the feet in line.*
3. *Bring the ankle bones together*
4. *Big toe joints touching.*
5. *Lift the inner arch of the feet.*

So, which of these instructions is right?

Clearly, for me, they cannot all be, so does that make some of the instructions wrong? What I am suggesting is that all of them are right or wrong depending on the person who is receiving the instruction. The risk we may run is that we begin to consider that there is a correct way to do an asana, and this immediately puts some of us in the position of failing.

Let me give you an example. A dear friend of mine is tremendously strong, but his body type and the work he has done all his life means that his feet turn out. He has what is sometimes referred to as ten to two feet. If he is asked to comply with any of the instructions above, it's simply not possible, and the effort of attempting it is extremely uncomfortable for him. So, does that mean he cannot do Tadasana?

What nonsense. He stands tall. He is the picture of strength and uprightness. People would give their right arm to be able to stand as he does. And yet those five instructions brand him as a failure. It's mad, is it not?

Let's take an anatomical look at the feet. The accepted mid-line of the foot is a line running from the second toe over the top of the foot to meet the shinbone. Try drawing a line on your feet, but ensure that you do not do as I did and use a permanent marker. (It took me a week to get it off).

In a world where everything has a correct position, then these mid-line lines that you have put on your feet might be parallel with one another, (Tadasana Feet). However, although we may accept the position of the mid-line of the feet themselves, that does not necessarily mean that the lines must both point in the same direction. The one thing we can say for certain about the human body is that it is NOT symmetrical. In fact, it is totally asymmetrical. No two bits are attached or behave in a symmetrical way.

Just look at the 3 sets of feet below, and then ask yourself which of the feet are right and which are wrong.

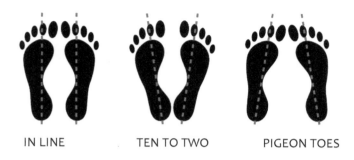

IN LINE   TEN TO TWO   PIGEON TOES

Hopefully, you may come to the conclusion that they are not right or wrong, just different.

Here is an interesting thought; the three types of feet shown above show symmetrical feet, as both feet are mirror images of one another. However, we know that we are not symmetrical, therefore, no one will have feet that are an exact mirror image. So, how many combinations might we have? At a quick count, I have identified maybe 15 combinations and that is without degrees of alignment.

If we take a conservative estimate and consider that the variation from straight-ahead feet to toes in and toes out is 10 degrees either way, then that's 20 degrees in total. If we multiply this up with different combinations that's 15 times 20 which gives us 300 possible natural/normal alignments of the feet. So, any alignment instruction given by any tutor as the correct one only has a one in 300 chance of being right.

Here is an example that I know exists as it is mine.

I cycle on a spin bike every day and have noticed that my right heel turns in a little and occasionally touches the crankshaft. It never hurts for it simply brushes it. The other foot, however, is nowhere near the crankshaft. Interesting. One person. Two feet. Both put on differently. How relevant may this be to every standing asana I do?

With this in mind, why would we attempt to fight the natural construction of the body, and a lifetime of acquired activities that make our posture what it is? It cannot be sensible to have to fight to make our feet fit a mould of what is proposed to be RIGHT by someone who knows little or nothing about an individual's personal physical construction.

I believe that inside all of us is an inherent limit to what we can achieve. If you are five feet 2 inches tall, then you are probably not going to make it into the Harlem Globetrotters, no matter how much you practise basketball.

However, if we lowered the height of the basket by 3 feet, who knows?

So, let's get realistic about asana and consider NOT how we can get into a posture, but instead, consider how we can wrap the posture around us. You would not, after all, consider getting into a coat for someone five feet tall if you were 6 feet 6. So why do it with asana?

Okay, so we now have got our feet right in Tadasana.

So where do we go from here?

Tall or mountain posture; this suggests that the actions we are reaching for are upwards towards the heavens. So, the operative word is UP. How can we encourage this action?

Well, if my wife Be is correct, and I believe she is, then every activity or thought that we have has the whole of the rest of the body listening in. So, if we say 'up' and carry out an activity that is up, the rest of the body might want to join in.

I would like to consider an instruction from my Iyengar days – *"Pull up on the kneecaps and thighs"*. I always found this less than comfortable, as it locked things up instead of freeing them.

If, however, we consider this to be a suggestion of an upward movement of the fronts of the legs, then the instruction and the action suggests UP, just what we want in Tadasana; rising up from a firm base.

While we are here, let's perhaps take a survey of what is happening so far. If I take a look, I can see and feel that with the instruction above, the inner arches of my feet have lifted. Interestingly, mula bandha has appeared too. What?? Just for lifting the kneecaps and thighs?

What I have also noticed is that I have a shadow of Uddiyana bandha. What about you?

With Uddiyana quietly active, it restricts the downward movement of the diaphragm to some extent and breathing moves towards being more mid and upper chest than normal. UP we go again. If we are tending towards mid and upper chest breathing, then add another instruction, *"lift the sternum, lift the collar bones"*. UP is again reinforced; and to an extent, a shadow of Jalandara bandha has appeared too.

If we allow the neck to be relaxed, and still send the message of UP, just maybe, Be is right and the whole body has been listening and joining in. Perhaps taking the first step towards levitation?

Now, let's take a look at the arms. Are our arms relaxed or active? One of the instructions I have been given has been "palms to the sides of the legs"; sort of at attention.

What if, just like our feet, our arms are not put on the same way? We are back to forcing the two arms to be the same. Why on earth would you do that?

See the picture below. These are my arms at rest; it's just the way they are put on.

I am quite happy with them and can find no good reason to twist one so they look the same.

Now, not only are we in a Tadasana that is right for each of us, but we have also introduced bandha without actually trying to do them.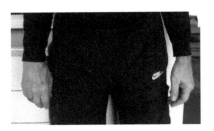

What do you think?

CHAPTER 2

Urdva Hastasana

Raised Hands pose

Urdva Hastasana, simply put, is Tadasana with the arms reaching upwards.

However, I would like to pose a question to you. How do we take the arms upwards? If there are different ways, does one particular approach make a difference? I will ask you to try two different approaches, and for you to enquire if the end result feels different.

We have just played with Tadasana and have considered that its driver has been 'upwards'. We mentioned earlier that the arms rest quietly by our sides, so let's add 'upwards' to the arms.

How should we take them up?

1. From Tadasana, with the arms at the side of the body, take the arms out to the sides, making a big semicircle until the fingertips point upwards. That's Urdva Hastasana.

Ask yourself how it feels and where your attention is.

2. From Tadasana, with the arms at the side of the body, bring the palms of the hands to the ears, that's 'upwards'. Now drive the hands straight up. That's Urdva Hastasana.

Ask yourself how it feels and where your attention is.

With both these approaches, we achieve Urdva Hastasana. What you have simply done is to enquire if the posture feels the same. If it does, that's fine. If it doesn't, that's fine too.

What we have done is to recognise that there is more than one way to attain a position, and made a decision for each individual based on enquiry.

With this simple experiment, we are being true to the principle that the Kalama Sutra expounds.

After investigation, believe that which you yourself have tested and found reasonable, and is for your good and that of others.

I wonder, has Urdva Hastasana been waiting quietly in Tadasana for you to discover it?

CHAPTER 3

Utkatasana

Chair pose

Here is an asana that follows Urdva Hastasana naturally.

From Urdva Hastasana, still thinking 'upwards', bend your knees. The knees go forward, and the butt tends to move back. Although the height of the asana has lowered, the reaching is still 'upwards'.

As if by magic, Utkatasana has appeared.

Now, here is an interesting question to consider. When we bend the knees in Urdva Hastasana, clearly, we are leaving Urdva Hastasana behind. So, when we bend the knees, does this mean that Utkatasana is now the asana?

The reason I ask you to consider this is that often I have heard mention that we will move through stages to the FINAL posture.

So, is there a point at which bending the knees in Urdva Hastasana is NOT Utkatasana, and that the body has to be at a certain position before we are IN the asana?

If this is the case:

What angle do the knees need to be bent to?
What angle must the upper body be at in relationship to the legs?
What angle must the arms be at?
Where must the gaze be?

We could ask a myriad of questions in an attempt to define Utkatasana, but if we go back to the outset, we can see again that only certain people can achieve the so-called RIGHT position; and anyway, who says what is RIGHT?

We need to consider that the asana should be about success for all. Setting so-called correct positions for limbs makes the attainment exclusive, when it should be inclusive.

Take a look at the stick people shown below. Two of them have been constructed from photos of well-known yoga practitioners and one is a common posture that I observe in my travels.

Now, ask yourself, which one is RIGHT?

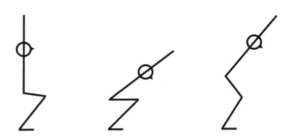

The one in the middle is only attainable if you have long calf muscles that enable the heels to maintain contact with the floor. So, let's ask, must the heels be in contact with the floor before we can define the posture? If you raise the floor under the heels, then everybody can go deeper into the squat. Is this okay?

I believe it would be fair to say that your choice or ability to perform any of the shapes shown above, or anything in between them, will be defined by your anatomy.

The floor itself will not alter, but your attachment to it may alter if you use blocks, wedges or even high-heeled shoes.

If this asana is defined by particular angles of the body, (the supposed correct way), then, for some of us, it will only be possible with the aid of props.

Surely it must be better to find your own perfect asana, working to *your* maximum, not someone else's.

Hopefully, you may come to the conclusion that these approaches or shapes are not right or wrong, just different.

If the practice of yoga asana is about the BALANCE between strength and flexibility, then can we also perhaps begin to stop being constricted by what we are told is RIGHT, and instead, consider what is RIGHT for each individual. This will allow us to return to the practice of fitting an asana around the individual, rather than fitting the individual into an asana.

If we wished, we could find examples of this in every asana that exists.

How often, as a student, do you simply carry out the instructions from the tutor without asking why? Well, some tutors may tell you (and this is from personal experience), *"Just get on with the practice and stop asking questions"*. Or *"I know it feels strange but just do it anyway; you will get used to it"*. Or *"Because this is the right way to do it"*. Or *"If you don't wish to carry out the instructions, it will be better if you leave"*. Or *"You are not trying hard enough; go into the beginners' class in the next room"*. Or *"You may have practised in a different way, but not in this class"*. Or *"Your hands are pointing in the wrong direction"*. The list is sadly quite long.

I am reminded of a comment from Billy Connolly when he was informed that he was doing something wrong. His reply, in a very strong and mildly aggressive Scottish accent, was, *"Oh, is that right then?"* Go Billy.

We could ask who knows the answers? Well; they may be answers for one, but they may not be yours. I am suggesting that a tutor should not be teaching students what they deem to be right, *(nor should the student just follow it blindly)*. The tutor should be offering paths to find what is right for each student. The tutor, without taking a view from somewhere else, cannot know with any certainty whether they are right or wrong, and should consider other views, knowing for sure that in the future those views may change; and that what is the truth now, is not THE truth, only A truth.

Here is a question for you. Should you only practice one type of yoga, one school, one approach, or should you investigate others?

Let us take a quote from Patanjali's yoga sutras (1-32) (1) where he suggests the value of "Not digging too many shallow wells, but to dig deep in one." This approach can, of course, be very valuable, for one of the keys to learning is not to flit about from one fad to the next, but neither do we want to dig so deep that eventually, we cannot see any light but that from the teacher's torch.

I am not suggesting that you question out loud every instruction that your tutor gives you, but rather to question the effect that an instruction has on you personally. Consider and make any adjustments that your body requires so that it feels right, and perhaps enquire of the tutor in a reasonable place and time. Students ask questions all the time in my classes. It never alters or affects the session negatively, but on the contrary, it is often a question that other souls had been thinking about and are glad that someone has asked. Oh yes, by the way, it keeps the tutor on their toes too.

Reference

(1) Desikachar, TKV, (1995) The Yoga Sutras of Patanjali; Affiliated East West Press

CHAPTER 4

Parvritti Utkatasana
Revolved Chair pose

Here is another asana that follows Utkatasana with some ease – Parvritti Utkatasana.

If we stay in Utkatasana, then we simply twist to one side or the other, move the arms to the prescribed position and, hey presto, we are in the posture. Sounds straightforward enough, but hasn't really allowed for much enquiry.

So, let's go back to Tadasana and consider if we should do Utkatasana first and then twist as above, or if we should twist first, then bend the knees and tip forward. You will end up in approximately the same place, but the journey that you have taken has been different and encourages questioning. How did I get to the same place but by a different route?

Well, it's no different than any journey we make take. If I were to go to London from Strood in Kent, I could go by car, or train, or coach, or walk, or bike. Each different mode of transport would take me on a different route and allow me to see and perceive the journey from a different point of view. Yet, whichever route I chose, I would still arrive in London. So, no one way is right; just different.

Okay, back to the asana. If we carry out the two possible approaches suggested above, we then ask the question 'where do the arms go'?

If your feet are together, which was the instruction I received during my career, I suggest we need to ask why.

I actually asked, and was given the following answer. *"As the right arm goes to the outside of the left leg, it puts pressure on the knee as we rotate against that knee to increase the twist, and it is the strength of the two legs together that allows the knee to be protected."*

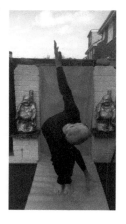

Sounds alright, so I ask, 'Why are we putting the right arm or hand to the outside of the left leg'? *"Because that's the way it's done,"* was the reply.

Elephant's Child asks: "Why does one hand have to be outside the opposite leg?"

If you need a lever to increase the twist, might it not make more sense to work on twists so that a deeper twist can be achieved in this variation of an asana?

Why can't the two arms be in the gravity line at half-past twelve, rather than at five to five or even ten to four? Or why not get some assistance from the tutor and a few mates and go for fifteen minutes to three?

The reality of the matter is that it's only books that say that the hand needs to go outside the leg. This then becomes the "right way" to do it. "Not always so" (1) says zen master Shunryu Suzuki.

So, let's have another look. If we get rid of the idea that the feet must be together in Tadasana and that the hand or arm does not have to go to the outside of the opposite leg, we can then observe that damage to the knee cannot arise. This is so as we are not using the legs as a lever to work against. If the arm is between the legs, then the need for the feet to be together to protect the knee is removed.

Just have a bash at this way.

From your Tadasana, have the feet apart, roughly under the hips. Bring the arms to shoulder level, put the twist in first, then bend the knees and then tip forward. One arm goes up and the other goes down. It may look something like the picture.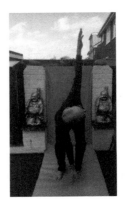

It is simply another approach, not right or wrong but different, just as you are different from every other person on the planet.

Remember, this is about enquiry. If, by practising both ways, you can explain to yourself why you are choosing a particular way, then all is well.

If, however, you are simply doing as you are told, then asana become nothing other than shapes as defined by a rule book. Enjoy.

Reference

(1) Suzuki S (2003) Not Always So: Practicing the True Spirit of Zen; Bravo

CHAPTER 5

Gravity line and Leverage

I wasn't sure where to place this section, as it is relevant to some extent to all asana. However, it is the next asana that we will be looking at (Uttanasana) where both gravity line and leverage are at play in both aspect and approach.

First of all, let me apologise if I am teaching you to suck eggs, but the importance of these two aspects of movement is, in my view, a prerequisite to both ease and safety in how we enter the activity.

Gravity line.

The gravity line is the line that runs through our body, enabling us to stand with the minimum of effort. Move out of it, and the body will attempt to bring you back into the gravity line. This is because our body is on our side and wants life to be as easy as possible, despite the contortions that yogis get into.

Take a look at Tadasana below.

Red is the gravity or centre line of the body always acting downwards.

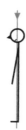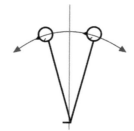

If we lean backwards or forwards from this position, the brain will instruct muscles either to bring us back to the centre, or, in extremis, to step back or forward to stop us from falling over.

In the real world, this activity of keeping us in the gravity line is used practically when we walk or run, for the reality of walking or running is, to put it simply, controlled falling over.

Have a bash at the suggestion below to experience this uncontrollable action.

Stand with your back to the wall, heels to the wall, and shoulders to the wall. Now, tip forward. How far can you tip forward before the feet grip the floor, the leg muscles tighten and eventually you have to step forward? The body has moved out of the gravity line and the brain wants to stop you from falling over, by instructing the muscles to act.

The picture below shows just how this happens in Utkatasana.

We can see that the head and the knees have moved forwards, and the butt has moved backwards to keep the body in the gravity line. It is keeping us balanced. We don't have to instruct these actions, they happen naturally.

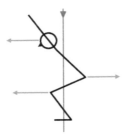

When we consider our next asana, Uttanasana, we will consciously use this natural action to enter and leave the posture, instructing and co-operating with the body, rather than fighting it.

Leverage

Leverage is the mechanical principle that states that as a weight at the end of a lever (our arm, for example) moves away from the centre or gravity line of the body, its apparent weight increases.

Let us see how this works with a practical example. Get yourself a can of beans or tomatoes or potatoes or soup. It doesn't matter what is in it. Say it weighs 1 kilo.

Put the can in a bag with handles to make it easy to grip. Hold the can in the bag by your side.

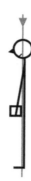

See how long you can hold it for before the arm becomes tired. It will probably be a fairly long time, and you may want to save your precious time and give up when you feel like it. Suffice to say that you will find this exercise fairly easy. I suggest we will feel little or no strain as the can in the bag is in gravity line and weighs just 1 kilo.

Now, take the can in the bag, and hold it at arm's length in front of you

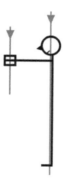

You may notice straight away that it feels heavier. I would suggest that you cannot hold it out there for as long as you could when it was by your side.

Why is this?

Clearly, the can has not increased in weight, but it feels much heavier.

This is because the distance between the can and the centre or gravity line of the body has increased.

What we get is something called Foot Pounds; in new terminology, Centimetre Kilos. This apparent weight is calculated by measuring the weight of the can multiplied by the length of the lever.

In this case, the lever is my arm, which is 65 Centimetres x 1 Kilo = 65 Centimetre Kilos.

For although the can itself still only weighs I kilo, its apparent weight has increased because we have multiplied the distance from the centre line to the can (65 centimetres) by the weight of the can (1 kilo).

However the calculation works, the most important thing for us to remember is that anything that is away from the centre line of the body becomes heavier and heavier which puts greater strain on some part of the body.

It will be useful to consider this as you enter your practices.

CHAPTER 6

Uttanasana

Standing Forward Bend

How do we define Uttanasana?

It's a standing forward bend and is clearly related to the previous asana that we have considered. In fact, it starts where we began, in Tadasana, and folds forward.

To some extent, this gives us carte blanche to do anything we like really, as long as we are standing and tipping forward to some degree.

We can ask

Is there an amount of folding forward that defines it?

If there is, where is it?

Is it defined by a person who can fold themselves into a small suitcase?

Is it defined by an Olympic gymnast?

The reality is that it is defined by what your particular body can do when at its maximum.

Let's ask a few more questions about aspects of the asana.

Must the legs be straight or can they be bent?

Where are the hands and arms placed?

What is the correct feet position?

Above are just three of the possible questions relating to what the asana may look like. Your guess or effort is as good as mine as to which one is RIGHT.

What we can say is that none of them is right; only a particular person's view of them makes it right.

It is most important to remember that the perfect posture does not actually exist, because we would then need to know what makes it perfect or right. We could have tutors with score cards like on Strictly Come Dancing. In the world of dancing, whether ballroom, Latin or modern, there are set rules on what is right and what is wrong. However, even with these rules, the judges still disagree with one another. I rest my case.

In the previous chapter, we considered the gravity line and how it runs through the body, and how our body works towards keeping us in line, so that standing and moving are as effortless as possible. We considered that if we move away from the centre line, the body will compensate and move a different bit of us to keep us balanced.

So, with this in mind, let us consider one approach and see what questions it asks us.

From Tadasana, reach up to Urdva Hastasana, and then fold forward at the hips.

As the torso moves forward, the butt moves back, and with the arms reaching away, we fold forward and down. With this action, we have our first question.

Why are the arms straight up to start? Remember leverage? With the arms reaching away, the weight of them multiplies and puts greater strain on the spine. Why would we do this? What advantage does this give us? Does it make the fold forward easier or more intense?

I believe it is taught like this because it's always been done this way. If you have taken a balanced view and practise, and can gain value from taking this action, then that's excellent, but I am suggesting that you don't just do it because it is what you have always done.

Instead, start again with the hands on the hips, take the forward fold, and ask yourself what the difference is.

Okay, let's come back to the beginning, and instead of tipping the torso forwards, instead, push the butt backwards, and observe the torso going forwards to counter the backward movement. You will still end up going into the asana, but is it different? It's your choice and it's an investigation, not an order.

Here is something worth experimenting with. If we consider anatomically where the majority of our weight is carried in the feet, it's the heels. Over 60% of our weight goes down through the heels. So, if you take more weight into them, the body will naturally recognise it and tip the torso forwards. Hey ho, the heels have begun Uttanasana.

We need to ask ourselves if straight legs define the asana. For example, if the legs are not straight, is it not Uttanasana?

Let's instead go back to Utkatasana, but this time with our hands on our hips and take another approach. Instead of working to keep the torso as upright as possible, and the abdomen moving away from the thighs as we do with Utkatasana, this time, we fold farther forward, keep the knees bent and rest the abdomen on the thighs. Clearly, this is not Utkatasana as we have folded forward, so is it Uttanasana? I would suggest that if it is your intention, then it is Uttanasana. Also, with this approach, we can observe that Uttanasana has appeared from Utkatasana, demonstrating an inherent link between the two asana.

There is a great advantage with abs to thighs, and that is that the spine is protected. If we look at the posture done by very flexible people, you will find that even with straight legs, their abs rest against the thighs.

So, the question becomes, 'Are we aiming for straight legs or abs to thighs and which of these define Uttanasana?' What do you think?

Okay, back to abs to thighs. Wrap your arms around your thighs, so that they cannot part from the abs, and now work towards straightening your legs. Concentrate on keeping abs to thighs; do not be concerned about how straight the legs are. Let your hamstrings be restricted by abs to thighs, not by your back.

If, like me, your legs do not completely straighten, it's still a fine Uttanasana, defined by our body's ability to get to its maximum. If we set the rules for the asana in stone, then most yogis would not be able to do it.

Forget the pictures in books where the legs are straight, for that may not be you. Just work to your measure. Play around; don't let the experts tell you what is right for you. You are the expert where your body is concerned.

Let the rules be set in blancmange, not stone.

Here is another question when we begin in Tadasana. Should we curl the spine forward allowing the back muscles to lengthen and close the chest, or begin with a shadow of a back arch, what might be referred to as lifting the sternum, with the back muscles engaged and encouraging a lengthening of the front of the body?

Aha, yet another question. Has lifting the sternum engaged the back muscles, or has the sternum lifted because we engage the back muscles? Just asking.

As we work deeper into the asana, eventually, the front of the body will close. Our enquiry should be, do we close it first or last? We need to experiment and experience both methods to find out which method works best for us as individuals.

As upright apes, we have a tendency to close our chest, so the back muscles naturally lengthen habitually. Ask yourself, as you sit at a computer or desk or workbench, are you sitting upright or slouching?

The next time you are approaching an old person's home, you may see a relevant road sign, a stooped, round-backed couple, much shorter than they used to be, for that is what life tends to do to us as we age.

Personally, I would rather be upright and taller, not shorter and rounded, but that's just my personal preference. What is yours?

I would like a pound for every time I have been told, "I can't touch my toes". If this were the case then most of us would not be able to tie our shoe laces. So, we bend the knees, then it's easy. Uttanasana is like that; bend your knees to do the asana then straighten them later, or never maybe.

CHAPTER 7

Parsvottanasana
Side Stretch pose

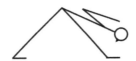

On the face of it, this asana looks a bit flash, but really, it's just a simple forward bend (Uttanasana, our previous asana) that has mucked about with the arms, and taken a step backwards. Let's ignore the arms for the moment and look at them later in this chapter.

For many years, before I started thinking for myself, I carried it out as below:

Stand in Tadasana, facing the long side of the mat.
Jump or step the feet wide apart.
Turn one foot in a bit (the back foot) and the other foot (the front foot) out 90 degrees.
Now swivel so that the torso faces over the front leg.
Fold over the front leg.

What on earth is all that about? A simple forward bend has had a twist incorporated into it and has left that back leg twisted to get the hips to face forward.

Why has this been done? For surely there are plenty of asana that incorporate a similar action? So, why use it with this one? Could it be because it's always been done like that?

Let's come back to Tadasana.

If we face the short side of the mat, we already have the hips facing the direction we want without twisting.

Do we, from this position, step forward or backwards? I don't mind, but prefer to step backwards. What I would say is that whether you choose to step backwards or forwards, your attention should be on the back foot. It is my view that the back foot is the anchor of the posture, keeping the whole of the foot in contact with the floor.

At first, I liked to have my feet really far apart because I was sure it was better and certainly looked good.

However, the back foot either lost contact with the floor or swung out to allow the greater distance I wanted to have for looking good. What I achieved, in fact, was to put the twist in the back leg, in other words, back to the original alignment I mentioned above. What for?

So, my answer to the first question, "How far do you step back?" depends on how far you can get the feet apart yet still keep them in the Tadasana feet position and well in contact with the floor.

You could ask why we need to step back or forwards very far at all. No one has ever given me an answer that has any rationale to it.

So, we can set a principle that will allow us all to find our own foot position.

As parsvottanasana is a forward bend, it makes sense to have the feet pointing forwards, pointing the way to go.

Step one foot back, still keeping the back foot in your own Tadasana foot position.

Ensure that the back heel is well in contact with the floor when you do, and do not allow the heel to kick in. Hey presto, all we need to do now is fold forward.

Get a feel for how the feet behave. Give this a go.

Start by facing the wall and come into Parsvottanasana. Use the wall, not just to give support, but to push against and drive the weight into the back foot. The calf muscles might be talking to you when you do this. Again, I am suggesting that awareness of this activity at the back of the posture enables the forward movement.

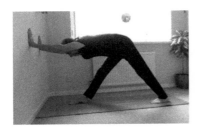 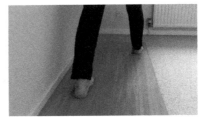

Feet in "tram lines"

With the feet set, keeping the back heel strongly in contact with the floor, bend the front knee a bit and see if you can bring the front thigh and abdomen together.

With them as close together as possible, begin to straighten the front leg which will encourage the movement to push into the anchored back foot. How interesting; we have a forward bend appearing that is going backwards.

If you are comfortable here, you may take the hands to the floor or onto the shin; use blocks to raise the floor to your hands if preferred. That's it, legs and body done.

Once you are at ease with the legs and the forward bend bit, we can consider doing the posture without the initial wall aspect, but adding the arm positions before entering the posture.

Ask yourself what works anatomically best for you and encourages the chest to open.

Below are some suggestions that allow us to find what suits each individual body and recognises that not all of us can achieve what the book says.

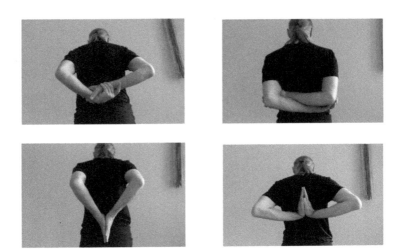

Try this one if you want to intensify the practice

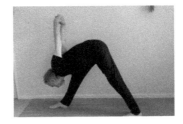

Please understand that I am not saying that any other approach is wrong; they are different but that's all they are.

If yoga is an investigation into the self and asana are an investigation into the nature of our bodies and you have a preference for one method or another, then that's great, but make sure you know why you are doing it. Investigations begin with questions, and "Because I like it" or "That's the way my teacher tells me to do it" is not really an answer.

CHAPTER 8

Trikonasana

Triangle pose

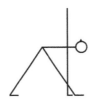

Is this Trikonasana? It looks like it to me. So, is it a side bend? Or is it a forward bend and a twist? Or is it something in between? These were questions I was first asked by Pete Blackaby, and little was I to know that this question would trigger the rest of my investigations into the nature of the postures. So thanks, Pete. Okay, 'Trikona' means triangle, so this asana is a posture of triangles. Nowhere does it state categorically that this needs to be done with open hips, nor as a forward bend with a twist, nor anything else really. These views are simply one person's interpretation of the asana, and how to be in it. It does not make any of them right.

Let's look at building Trikonasana and start from the feet.

Some tutors are quite prescriptive about where the feet may be placed and may say 2 feet apart or 4 feet apart. What we need to ask is, who does this instruction apply to? Me, or someone who is 4 feet 9 tall, or someone who is 6 feet 8 tall? Again, we are in the field of everything is right or wrong but not all the time nor for everyone.

So, the distance apart is different for everybody; that's solved that one.

Now, at what angle do we place the feet? Take a look at the picture and let's consider the foot positions. The centre line represents the body's midline; the outer lines represent hip width.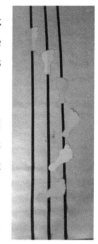

Shown are foot positions that I have been instructed to carry out by respected, knowledgeable yoga tutors from different schools and different approaches, except one, (my one) because it really works well for me.

Considering ORANGE feet; heel of front foot in line with inner arch of back foot.

My first question is, "Why are we standing on a tightrope?" Well, it is suggested that this alignment is the best position for working towards opening the hips. Okay, so if opening the hips is the plan, then why is the back foot turning in?

If the plan is to open the hips, then surely the back foot needs to turn out. But we are told to turn it in. Why?

If we want to open the hips, why on earth don't we turn both feet out? I have tried it and it's not that comfy, nor does it encourage a side bend much. It seems to me that to do the posture in this way compromises too many activities. Do have a go and make your own mind up.

Okay, back to the beginning. "Turn the left foot out. Turn the right foot in." These instructions give direction, and as both feet are moving to the left, it seems fair to believe that the posture is moving left.

Now we are told, "Rotate the right thigh outwards to open the hips." Again, this is an instruction I have received hundreds of times.

So, we have the right foot turning in, and the leg at the hip turning out. Sitting between these two opposing actions is the knee joint, a joint that primarily is a joint of flexion. It does not like rotating. Yet the two forces that we have applied to the knee are opposites, and so some degree of rotation is forced at the knee joint. Why would you do that?

Of course, the ankle joint will take on some of the work, but the fact remains that we have two opposing actions in the same leg.

What about BLUE feet?

Similar, except we have avoided the tightrope a bit. The instructions that I received were as above, so the same activity at the knee is present.

What about GREEN feet?

Here, the actual approach to entering the asana is different. We still start from hip-width apart Tadasana, but this time, we simply step the right foot back, keeping the feet roughly the same width apart as they were. There is a tendency to step the foot to the mid-line; avoid this; just step straight back. My friend Hugh Grainger suggested the gap between the inner borders of the feet should be at least enough to fit two tracks of

Hornby Double O gauge (that's model railway jargon. A Scalextric track also fits the bill).

The step back is not huge, as we are not attempting to get the feet miles apart; it's a reasonable step back. Now, fold forward at the hips about halfway. Once there, rotate to the right and place the left hand inside of the left foot.

Take the right hand skywards, and look over your right shoulder if the neck feels good.

Wahoooo, Trikonasana?

You can see with this approach that there is no attempt to open the hips, yet it clearly demonstrates the construction of triangles that, to my mind, makes it Trikonasana.

All the stuff above is from acknowledged experts and I have had a bash at all of them and really enjoyed the experience, and still do sometimes. So, try all three and enjoy which way suits you best. This way, you will experience what you are doing to your body and why you are doing it.

What about old PINK feet?

This is the approach I most enjoy for MY anatomy.

From Tadasana, facing the side of the mat, step the feet apart.

Turn the left foot out 90 degrees. Turn the right foot in strongly, (almost facing forward).

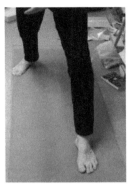

Raise the arms to shoulder level with the palms facing down.

We have turned both feet to the left, so the message the body is receiving is to rotate to the left. Now let us encourage this action with the pelvis. Drive the right hip forward and draw the left hip back. This will encourage the torso to move towards the left.

Ensure that the shoulder girdle stays on its original plane so that the pelvis is rotating under the stationary shoulder girdle.

With the actions suggested above, to some extent, the torso is automatically being drawn to the left, so just follow it, reaching away to the left and keeping the chest open.

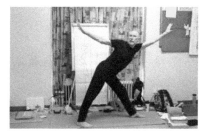

This action of reaching away (not down) will encourage the left side of the torso to lengthen, maintaining length on the underside of the body, and resisting the top side of the torso's desire to arch up.

Eventually, you will not be able to reach any farther away, so the arm/torso will have to go down, finding the inside of the left leg or floor or block. Voila, Trikonasana.

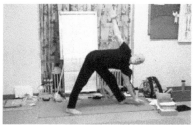

Here is another question relating to Trikonasana, but this time, to the eventual hand position.

Why, in some instructions, is the hand taken to the outside of the front foot?

No matter what foot alignment we may take, the hand to the outside of the foot will never be in the centre or gravity line. What can happen is that the top arm is thrown farther back in an effort to open the chest, as shown right.

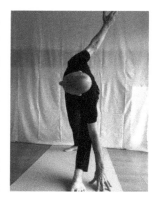

Or the arms are not in gravity line at all because the hand to the outside of the foot closes the chest.

My view will always be that best gravity line alignment is the first goal of the asana. What is your view?

This instruction of hand to the outside of the foot has become almost biblical, immaterial of a student's ability to practically reach it. Often, it is suggested that we use blocks to attain it. Well, it certainly helps; but why not work towards alignment first, and then, as we develop, work towards hand to the outside of the foot? The question this raises is, "What is it that makes the final posture of Trikonasana about hand placement?" (My view is that it is not about that).

If, instead, we place the hand on the inside of the foot (the centre line of the body), it in no way restricts openness in the chest, but actually encourages openness and alignment.

If you cannot place the hand on the outside of the foot with ease, then you need to ask yourself why you are doing it. What is this hand outside instruction all about? What is its value to you? And even if you can do it, why are you doing it?

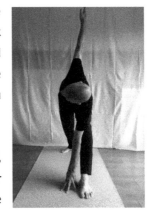

Don't just take my word for it, try it yourself, and whatever you decide will be right (for you). This is not to say that for the more supple amongst us, outside is wrong, but by the same standard, don't let it be the correct or ultimate position either.

Oh yes, by the way, do the same to the other side, or you may end up walking in gentle circles to the left without ever knowing it.

Chapter 9

Parvritti Trikonasana
Revolved Triangle pose

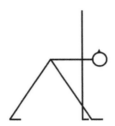

The stickman above claiming to be Parvritti Trikonasana actually looks exactly the same as Trikonasana. However, let's look at the differences.

With Trikonasana, the hand moves towards the same side foot (right hand to right foot, for example). With Parvritti Trikonasana, the hand moves towards the opposite foot (right hand to left foot, for example). These may be minor in describing, but a bit of a challenge in actually doing, for it is in the practice that the challenge comes, for now, we are rotating the pelvis AND the torso to achieve the hand position.

All the challenges that we considered for the back leg in Trikonasana are intensified in Parvritti Trikonasana. Remember, "Why are we opening the hips?"

In Trikonasana, as mentioned above, the right hand goes to the right foot (depending on what side you are doing), and the shoulder girdle remains facing forwards, above the rotating pelvis. The pelvis is putting a twist into the spine at the outset.

In Parvritti Trikonasana, to achieve opposite hand to foot then, the rotation needs to be encouraged, as it has to be greater. Do relook at the foot position in the previous section on Trikonasana and consider that, with the back foot facing more forward, it enables greater rotation.

So, from our legs apart position, we begin to drive the pelvis forward. Previously, in Trikonasana, we kept the shoulder girdle facing forward, but this time, as the pelvis rotates, we allow the torso to go with it. Eventually, of course, the pelvis will run out of room to rotate, and it is at this moment that the torso carries on the rotation, and allows the opposite hand and foot to meet.

So, in Trikonasana, the pelvis initiates the rotation in the spine (spinal rotation first); in Parvritti, the shoulder girdle joins in the rotation once the pelvis has stopped (spinal rotation last).

Once the rotation has gone as far as it can, the hand and foot move towards one another, and hey presto, Parvritti Trikonasana has appeared. What fun we are having.

Okay, let's go back to the hand positions we considered in Trikonasana. The challenge in Parvritti Trikonasana is clearly greater, so I would encourage you to consider again the biblical instruction of hand to the outside of the foot, and ask yourself, "Who says, and why do they say it, that this hand position is the correct eventual position?"

Take a look at the two pictures below and ask yourself:

Which one is best aligned?

Which one allows for greater ease of opening the chest?

They are both Parvritti Trikonasana.

But what one is right?

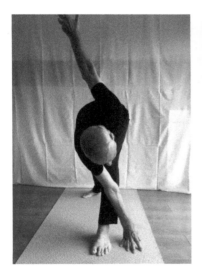 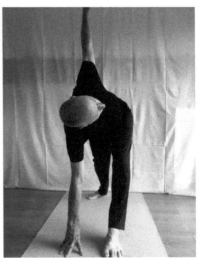

I don't know the answer to the last question, but I do know the answer to the first two.

What do you think?

CHAPTER 10

Prasarita Paddotanasana
Wide Leg Forward Bend

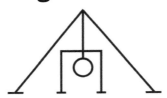

All that we considered in Uttanasana (standing forward bend) applies to Prasarita Paddotanasana, for the only difference is that the legs are wide apart. It is still a standing forward bend.

Our first question: How wide is wide?

It's the width apart that your legs can go that is reasonable for your body type. This doesn't mean that it should be easy, so sweet discomfort, not pain. But don't go beyond that which is reasonable. Remember, yoga is not a competition, but a series of activities that stretch and strengthen us physically and mentally.

As we take the feet and legs apart, the legs and the soles of the feet move out of the gravity line. So instead of the weight going straight through the ankle joint to the ground, the weight is either being driven outwards, where it lifts the inner arch of the feet and we lose full sole contact, and put a strain on the ankle joint,

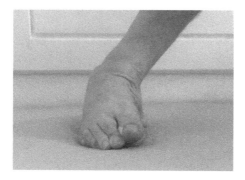

or the feet collapse inwards, again losing sole contact with the floor, and in this example, putting strain on the knee.

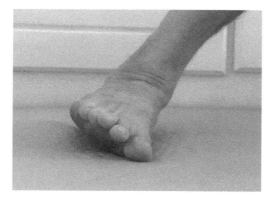

Or, as below, the sole of the foot is firmly in contact with the floor, setting an even base out of which the posture can appear.

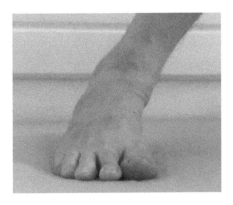

I am suggesting that any of the feet positions shown above are the results of how wide apart we set the feet.

So, ask yourself what is best for your feet and knees, and set the feet apart accordingly.

As with Uttanasana, when entering the asana, we need to consider how we can use as little effort as possible.

Now we are here, let us experiment with the weight on the feet and ask what happens as we move it about.

First, take the weight into the balls of the feet and fold forward; ask yourself what is happening and where you feel it as you go. Now, take the weight into the heels and fold forward; ask yourself what is happening and where you feel it as you go. If you feel a difference, that's the key, as now you can make an informed decision about what works best for you.

All of the above we have done with straight legs, so what happens when you bend the knees? Good old gravity line and the shifting of the centre of the body in space will assist and enable the posture to develop itself.

Take a look at the picture below.

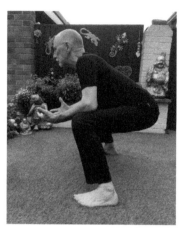

If we bend the knees, the torso just wants to go forward. If we now place our hands on the floor, is this the posture? Or are straight legs the posture, without hands to the floor? Is there a correct interpretation that categorically states when it is or isn't the posture?

If, from here, we bring our hands to the floor or to blocks and then straighten the legs, you will end up somewhere like me below. Can you see how the weight has shifted into the heels to maintain lightness in the upper body?

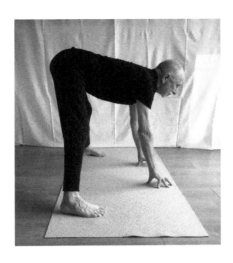

This is just me, and you are just you and equally correct.

If we approach the practice with straight legs, then the same can be achieved, simply by taking the butt backwards and the weight into the heels. This action encourages the torso to move forwards in response to the butt moving backwards. It's the old adage *'For every action, there will be an opposite and equal reaction'*. We are simply using this principle to get things done, working to the maximum by using the minimum.

Don't take my word for it; give it a go.

CHAPTER 11

Parsvakonasana

Side Stretch or Angle posture

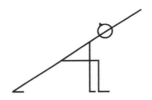

Side angle posture.

It poses some of the questions that Trikonasana does, but whereas Trikonasana (triangle) is based on the triangle shape *(its shape makes it very strong)*, Parsvakonasana does not have that attribute. For as the front knee bends to make the shape, the strength gained from a triangle disappears and sets the body a whole new set of considerations.

The posture consists of two geometric shapes below the waist; a triangle and a square (Red) filling the space.

The triangle's strength depends on there being three joined sides, and it can be seen that one of these sides is missing (black broken line)

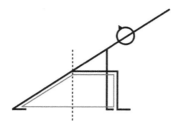

The square is also missing a side (black broken line) and even with 4 sides, a square is naturally deformable, and to maintain its integrity depends entirely on our physical strength.

So, when we bend the front knee, the square might not end up square, but as a diamond shape. All this is fine as long as we have good enough physical strength to maintain it.

Remembering that gravity operates downwards and that this force will put the most pressure on those areas that are unsupported either by muscular strength or skeletal integrity, so, in this instance, this area will be the rear knee, particularly if the back foot is turned in with the consequence that the force will be going through the side of the knee.

Let us remember this as we begin the asana.

Let us come to the start position as in Trikonasana, one foot out, the other one in (feet width as in Trikonasana, your choice), with balanced, firm contact of the feet with the floor.

Now, as we bend the front knee for Parsvakonasana to appear, the front knee goes forward. As this happens, the rest of the body listens to what is happening, and thinks, looks like everyone is going forward to a party, so let's all go too. Everyone wants to go, except the back foot, let's call him "Billy no mates". He actually quite likes it where he is, planted firmly and strongly on the floor at the back.

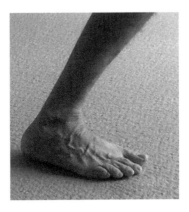

To enable Billy to go to the party, a couple of things might happen. The inner arch of the back foot may collapse, and the outer edge of the foot may rise from the floor.

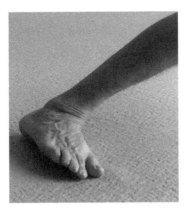

If this action happens, any support that the rear knee had has been removed, and gravity will drive down through the unsupported knee.

Instead, if we work with the rear foot in the first position above, then the rear foot can act as an anchor. Thus, we are operating from a position of strength and stability in the rear leg.

What this will do, however, is to restrict the degree to which the front knee can bend. What I am suggesting is that the bend of the front knee should be governed by the position of the back foot's contact with the floor, not by attempting to make any particular angle. Just play around with those two foot positions and ask yourself, what makes sense?

What may disappoint some of us is that we cannot get the hand to the floor, nor bend the front knee as far as the book or tutor tells us it should. Ah, what a shame.

If, instead, we concentrate on powering the outer edge of the back foot firmly down, it will enable the body to resist gravity's downward movement through the back knee and protect it. A firm rear foot will also restrain us from lunging forward in an effort to get our front knee at right angles to the floor. For we all know that 90-degree front knee and hand to the floor is the RIGHT position.

Or is it?

If we kick the 90-degree front knee and hand to the floor scenario firmly into touch and concentrate on a long straight line from the fixed outer edge of the back foot to the tips of fingers, we might end up with something like this.

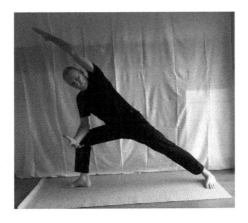

No, the front knee is not 90 degrees, nor is the hand to the floor, but this looks like Parsvakonasana to me. What do you think? Give it a try.

We now come to that old chestnut already considered in Trikonasana. Where do we place the hand – with or without blocks, inside or outside of the front foot?

Shown right is a position of the front knee that I have seen countless times during my yoga life in Parsvakonasana. It is not a position that the knee likes much, but is an often-inevitable position attained when we work in this asana.

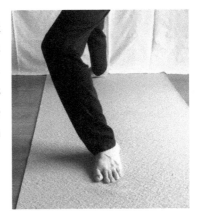

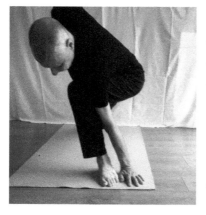

For most of us, if we place the hand to the outside of the knee, it is likely that many of us will end up with the front knee and leg as shown in this picture, firmly held in position by the arm, as we reach for the floor on the outside.

Why would you even think about putting the hand there?

As in Trikonasana, we could use blocks, but why not, as in Trikonasana, go for alignment first, and go for the hand outside position once you have perfected your alignment? Ask yourself, if you are going for the outside, why are you doing it?

Why not instead consider putting the hand on the inside, where it will actually keep the lower leg upright until enough strength and flexibility have been gained, so that if you want to attempt to place the hand on the outside, then you can.

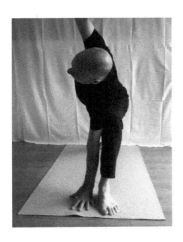

This raises the question, who says the hand must go outside? It is certainly not in the best anatomical position, and I cannot find a valid rationale for placing it there other than "that's where it goes". However, if you find a reason that clearly gives an anatomical benefit, let me know, please.

So, with the questions and answers that I have used in my practice, I have ended up with the shape alongside, and this looks all right to me. After giving it a try, what do you think?

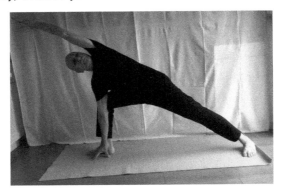

Another question-and-answer session relating to Parsvakonasana

Some years ago, by complete accident, I happened into a class with a guy called Howard Napper. He told us we were going to do Parsvakonasana and proceeded to get us all into a longish cat.

I thought, 'What's going on here? Is he mad? This is not the way it is done.'

However, my interest overcame my certainty, and I gave it a go.

We stepped one leg forward, both hands to the floor, toes of the back foot tucked under.

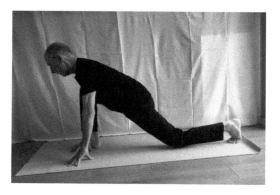

What???? Surely the whole sole of the back foot must rest on the ground, not just the ball of the foot. I knew that I had to turn the foot so that this could happen, disregarding Howard Napper's instruction 'toes of back foot tucked under'.

This man is losing his mind. I knew I was right. But being a little mad myself, I continued to follow the tutor's instruction and kept the toes of the back foot tucked.

Anyway, the madness continued.

With one hand inside of the front foot, we took the other one onto the lower back. Remember earlier we talked about the body going to a party? Surprise, surprise, the whole torso went too, and we ended up looking over our shoulder rotating the torso and opening the chest.

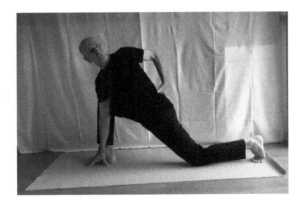

Now, although the torso has rotated, because the back knee is resting on the floor, the back leg's ability to rotate is minimal, so the heel has not swung in, but has remained in an upright position.

We now drove the back heel backwards. Concentrating on this backwards movement, I found that my knee rose of its own accord. Weird. Give it a try.

This led to me experimenting. So, instead of driving the heel back, I simply lifted the knee. What I found happened was that as the knee rose, so did the butt. So, instead of getting a straight top line, I ended up looking a bit like a camel; the one hump kind, a dromedary.

This suggested to me the "body going to a party" activity again. The body thinks if the knee is going up then let's all go up.

Meanwhile, I had noticed that when the heel was driven back, the knee simply straightened and the straight top line was maintained.

Try this activity yourself and see what your investigations say.

Now let's take a look at how we get the top arm to its place.

In the past, when I have worked with the top arm position, I always used to take the arm up and over to bring the upper arm alongside the ear. If we consider "body going to a party" again, then the listening body will hear 'up', and up it will go in concert with the arm. That's what happens with me, anyway. Have a go yourself.

So, try this approach instead. It's just a try. You don't have to agree with it, but it may give you some points to ponder.

Place the hand on the ear and drive the arm past the ear. Now we have an action of the back foot going back and the top hand going forward, lengthening from the centre:

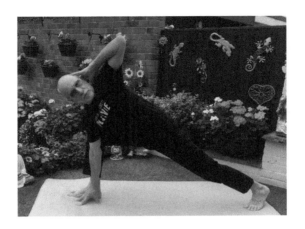

And ending up like this:

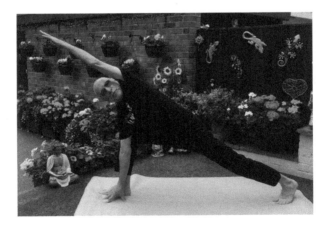

The major principle is still to take the action of the asana into the back foot. It's just that we have approached it from a different direction and the leg is in its anatomical, natural plane and the knee is never at risk. Wow, we have bonuses everywhere.

Of course, we have not rotated the back leg to open the hip, but as this is a posture of side lengthening, why do we need to rotate the leg and consequently open the hips to do the posture?

The pelvis opening is only someone's interpretation of what the posture is, and they have as much chance of being correct, or not, as anyone else does.

Play with all the ideas, and come up with the answers that are right for you. Enjoy.

CHAPTER 12

Parvritti Parsvakonasana
Revolved Side Stretch or Angle pose

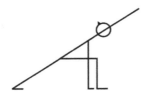

Remember the difference we looked at with Triangle and Revolved Triangle? Well, the same principles apply here

With the Side Stretch pose, the hand moves towards the same side foot (right hand to right foot, for example). With Revolved Side Stretch, the hand moves towards the opposite foot (right hand to left foot, for example). Again, minor in describing, but a bit of a challenge in actually doing.

The stickman above claiming to be Parvritti Parsvakonasana actually looks exactly the same as Parsvakonasana. It is in the practice that the test comes, for now, we are rotating the pelvis AND the torso to achieve the hand position, complicated by the fact that the front knee is bent.

We can dispense with all the info about feet and legs, as they are the same as for Parsvakonasana.

The real difference is that where in Parsvakonasana we have an open twist (rotating the chest away from the front leg), now we have a closed twist, where we rotate the chest towards the front leg.

Closed twists are always more challenging, as the front leg tends to get in the way of the rotation.

We could consider the two approaches that we did in Parsvakonasana –

1. foot in full contact with the floor;
2. ball of the foot to floor with heel raised.

However, as we are only really looking at the twisting aspect, I will dispense with running through them both again, as it is hand placement that we will be considering and questioning.

I will also dispense with detailed Q&A relating to hand position, and instead, simply offer two pics that you can investigate yourself.

This first one is hand to the outside. Ask yourself. If I attempt to take my hand to the outside of the foot, does it encourage natural alignment (knee over the ankle) or has it forced it into the centre and out of natural alignment?

If it has become out of alignment in your attempt to carry out this action, then ask yourself why you are doing it, and what advantage have you gained from it?

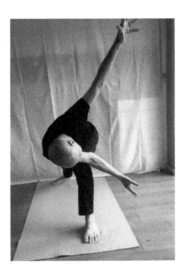

The second one is hand to the inside.

The knee has no twist in it and is on its natural anatomical plane, and the upper body has space into which it can rotate.

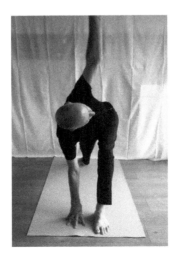

I would encourage you to play around with these positions and find out which works for you.

If you feel that the outside hand position is where you want to be, that's great after investigation. But do remember that it is not THE right place for it, only A place.

Investigate and enjoy.

CHAPTER 13

Virabhadrasana
The warriors

This next chapter has three asana in it, and I would ask you to consider it as you would watching or reading a play. A play is split into acts or parts. Alone, each act does not make the play. It is complete in its context, but you will need to read or see all the acts to understand the play itself.

I would like you to approach the warrior asana with the same thought in mind.

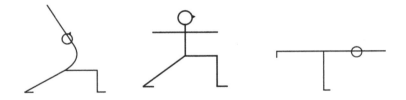

Warrior 1 is the Bow Warrior 2 is the Archer Warrior 3 is the Arrow

I am suggesting that we cannot have a warrior without a bow and arrow, so although these three items are complete in themselves, they only become valuable when combined. Does that make sense?

Virabhadrasana 1

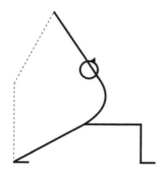

If we consider Warrior 1 above, it is clearly a bow shape, because if you tied a piece of string (Red) between the heel and the fingers and pulled it back, you would have a bowstring and something with which to fire your arrow.

Let's take a look at the construction of the posture.

Clearly, the hips are facing forwards. If they are not, why is that the case? If the hips don't face forward then we would need to put a twist into the asana. Then your question becomes, why would I need a twist to do a backbend? What do you think?

How do you take the feet apart? Do you (a) take the feet wide apart then turn to face over one leg, or (b) simply step forward or back? One of these puts a twist in the posture; the other doesn't.

You try.

First choose your back foot position, considering that you want the hips to face forward. Clearly, green feet are the ones that will most enable it, since all the others, to some extent, draw one hip back.

If you work with green feet, do you want the heel of the back foot on the floor or raised?

What are the advantages of a raised heel? Well, it allows you to have the feet much farther apart, and allows the front knee to bend more deeply. That's great if that's what you believe is the most important part of this asana, or simply that you look pretty good in it, and that's fine.

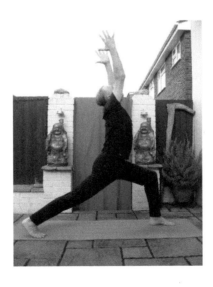

If, however, you work with the heel down, this will restrict how far your feet can be apart, and the amount that the front knee can go forward. You will not look quite so good in this version; however, you will look more like a bow.

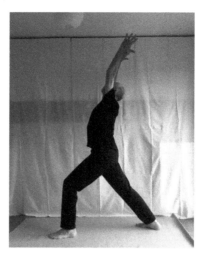

However, both of them are valid, just different.

I am going to suggest that you look at a bow, and ask a few questions of it.

Is it extremely curved before the bowstring is pulled? If not, why not?

Remember also that a bow is rigid and strong in the centre, as a weak or over-curved centre weakens the power of the bow. Further, consider that the power in a bow comes from the two ends. These are the most flexible parts of the bow and are what generate power when the bowstring is pulled. I believe this is where our effort and focus should be in this pose; the two ends of the bow.

So, ask yourself what sort of bow are you making; one that is awaiting the bowstring to be drawn, or one under bowstring tension? Both are good, and both are challenging in different ways. So, whatever your approach, always drive the back heel down, and take the hands up and back and allow the centre to be firm and strong, not bent.

Play around and see what you like.

I am going to consider the asana out of order, as I would like to get an arrow for our bow first. So, if that's okay with you, I will consider Warrior 3 now.

Virabhadrasana 3

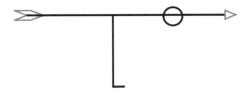

This asana is a balance, but it is only a balance because we have two legs. You see this posture is an arrow, and an arrow does not have a leg to balance on. Therefore, when we consider this posture, I would like you, as much as possible, to forget your standing leg and concentrate instead on the arrow bit.

The challenge is that we spend much of our time concentrating on balancing and possibly not enough time getting our arrow straight.

We are told that we need to make a T shape.

Please come back with me to the Battle of Hastings, where poor Harold lost his eye. I propose that Harold would never have lost his eye if the Normans had fired their arrows as in the stick man above, level with the floor. Those devious Normans, however, and any archer with any sense, fires the arrow upwards so that it goes farther and accelerates on its way down. This is common sense.

So why can't we have our arrow at any angle, as long as it is straight?

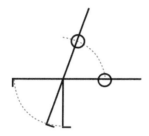

There is an advantage to this too, for it is much more possible to balance.

If you accept this suggestion, the next question is, how do we get there?

I know of two approaches, the first being from any wide leg posture, but let's use Trikonasana.

From Trikonasana, we turn the torso to face down, bring the arms to either side of the ears, bend the front knee and shift the weight carefully over the standing leg, then lift the back leg from the floor and come to balance.

Bit complicated, but it does get you there.

The second approach is one that I was inspired to try when I was at a yoga weekend away in a convent in Sussex.

Now the convent and the Nuns are an integral part of practising this way. Let me tell you the story.

The Nuns had a playground with an enormous adult size swing and a giant seesaw for four. Now the reasoning behind this was that the Nuns were all various sizes, and anyone who has been on a seesaw with someone of a different size will know that you either end up sitting on the ground, or are raised permanently to the heavens, and should the heavy person get off suddenly, you come crashing painfully down.

Not the Nuns, for, with two seats at either end, they could easily get the balance just right.

When I saw this, I thought Virabhadrasana 3! Why can't we swivel the torso and leg around the centre of the body, just like the seesaw and the Nuns?

So, I came into Tadasana, took my arms over my head, shifted the weight onto one foot and gently swivelled around the hip joint. Initially, I did not swivel to the T position, but why should I?

Although this posture will be called Warrior 3, for me it will always be 'Four Nuns on a Seesaw Asana'.

Give it a try and see what you think.

Virahadrasana, or Warrior 2

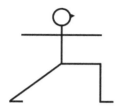

This asana is almost always done with the front knee bent; I don't know why, and nor does anyone else to my knowledge. However, I can live with it.

But, let us not forget that there is not an archer in the world that would bend their front knee when firing a bow and arrow. Nuff said.

Anyway, let us run with the bent knee.

Now I know that this asana can be approached from wide legs, and all that swivelling about stuff, but I would like you to consider it from the stepping back method just for today so that you can experience it. Don't give up your own method, but do have a think about other approaches.

Okay, from Tadasana, step back as far as is practical, and accept that the back foot is going to turn out a bit, however, remember that the back foot is the anchor and consider all the work we did on the strength in the back foot for other wide-leg postures.

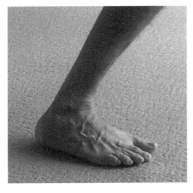 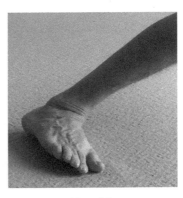

This   Not this

With the back foot well-anchored, bend the front knee to your maximum, not to the tutor's instruction. What you should have now is a nice firm base out of which to fire your bow and arrow. We consider the bits that will hold the bow and take straight arms to shoulder height.

Okay, let's rotate the front arm and make a fist (thumb upmost) as if holding a bow.

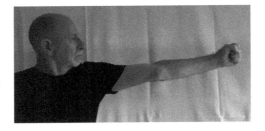

Now, bring the back hand forward, close to the front hand, as if reaching for the bowstring and its attached arrow.

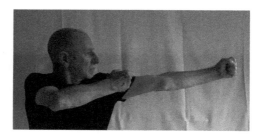

Now grasp the imaginary bowstring and arrow and bring it back strongly across the chest as if drawing the bow. This action ensures that the chest opens actively.

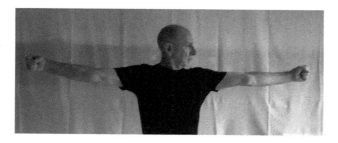

Keeping the chest open, aim the gaze forwards in the direction in which your arrow will fly.

Then open the hands and let the fingers reach strongly away from your centre.

Thus, the bow and arrow rest in space awaiting the moment of release.

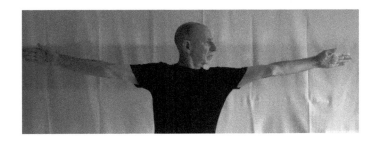

Okay, we have considered this three-part play. Let's get to the end and put the three acts together so that the warrior is complete. Not parts 1, 2 and 3, but the Warrior itself.

Something like this:

(Act 1)

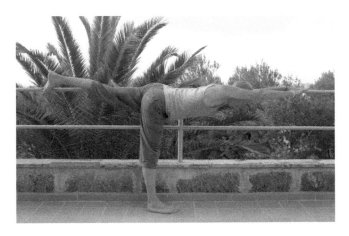

83

(Acts 1 and 2)

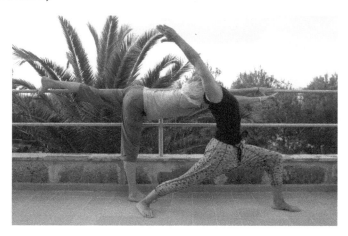

(Acts 1, 2 and 3)

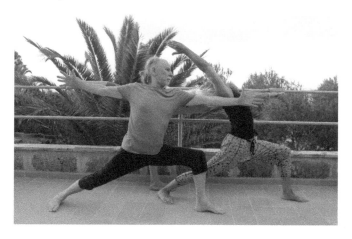

This next exercise will ask you to allow your mind to hold onto your Warrior creation.

Here we go:

Come to Tadasana. Step one leg back to your own measure. Take your arms over your head. Bend your front knee to your own measure. Reach up and back. Et voila, Warrior 1.

The Bow.

Hold this shape in your mind, and allow it to rest in the space you created.

Now shift the weight into the front foot, and, as you straighten the leg, coming into balance over it, swivel at the hips and the back leg lifts. Et voila, Four Nuns on a Seesaw; Warrior 3.

The Arrow.

Hold this shape in your mind, and let the arrow rest passively in the bow that you created earlier.

Soften the standing leg knee. Allow the raised leg to move back to the floor, bring the torso to upright and bend the front knee to your measure. Open the chest and bring the arms to shoulder level.

With the forward arm, grip the imaginary bow that you created previously. Bring the back arm to hold the imaginary bowstring and arrow, and draw it back across the chest.

And now, you are all the Warriors in one.

CHAPTER 14

Vrksasana

Tree

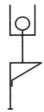

There really is not much to say about this posture as we are simply standing on one leg and taking the hands over the head.

The interesting bit is the raised leg: where do we place it (top of the foot, ankle, calf or thigh?) and how to get it there?

The two pics on the next page give placement possibilities.

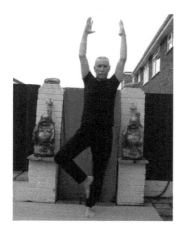 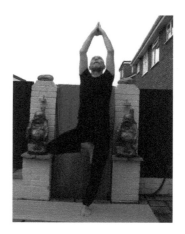

Or anything in between, as long as it is not on your knee.

So, now my question is, "What actions do we take to place the foot wherever is right for us?" In other words, what we are attempting to achieve?

Remember, we want the keep the pelvis facing forward.

Okay, here is one way.

Shift the weight onto the standing leg and rotate the other leg outwards so that the knee and the foot point away from the midline, using only muscular control.

Bend the knee, and place the sole of the foot on the inside of the standing leg.

If it rests on the knee joint, then place it on the calf. Or you may want to grab the ankle and yank it up above the knee. Be my guest, but ask yourself, "Why am I doing that?"

All great as long as at this point you are not encouraging the hips to open, for if you do, you will probably swing about on the hip joint, and instead of facing forward, you may find that the pelvis has rotated whilst the torso is facing forward.

Now you have added a twist to a balance. Why?

Here is another way.

Bend the right leg at the knee using only muscular control.

Take the knee away from the midline, stopping when the pelvis starts to move.

As above, place the sole of the raised foot wherever it rests, remembering the possibility of yanking the foot up. Remember to keep the hips facing forward and avoid swinging about on the hip joint.

If the pelvis has rotated whilst the torso is facing forward, you have added a twist into a balance. Why is that?

You have ended up in approximately the same position by two different routes.

Question: Which one is right? Answer: The one that suits you best.

With the pressure of the raised foot on the inner leg, there will be a tendency for the opposite hip to push out.

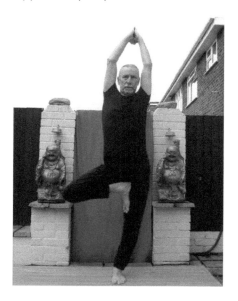

A bit snake-like.

Try bringing the attention to the hip joint of the standing leg, and draw it in to the centre line of the body. You may find that this action will drive the posture upwards, and bring the body into improved alignment.

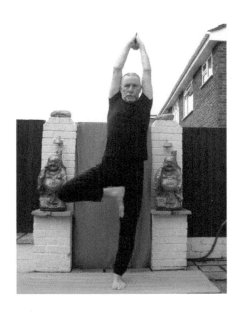

Straight.

Away you go.

Bonus

An enquiring journey

As I end this book, I would like to give just one example of how my questioning and thinking approach to asana can create interesting directions in which to travel.

I reflected how interrelated many asana are, and how we can flow from one asana to the other, and that there are loads of practices that do this, with Astanga Vinyasa, for example, the one that I have had most experience of.

Then my mind wandered to Rotation. Then Spirals and Circles, as you do. Suddenly, my thinking became somewhat expansive at this point, and this was how.

At a universal level, the universe is entirely driven by rotation. The earth is round and revolves on its axis. It goes around the Sun, which rotates around the Milky Way, which rotates around the – well, we could go on and on.

Likewise, on a micro level, we are built on rotation. At an atomic level, electrons revolve around a nucleus. Nuclei themselves are round, so again, we could go on.

Deoxyribonucleic acid, or DNA as we know it, is a series of linked circular spirals within us, and is the very building block of life.

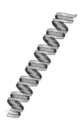

So, it seems that circles, spirals and rotation are movements that are inherent in our world and in our makeup. So, if this action is so inherent within and without, might it make sense to consider this in relation to our movements when practising our asana?

How often do we notice that lying quietly within each asana is rotation? Consider a standing forward bend (Uttanasana). Anatomically, it is flexion at the hips as the torso moves forward and down – however, this action is only made possible by the ability of the head of the thigh bone to rotate in the socket on the pelvis.

Even anatomical terminology (the position from which all movement is defined) is defined by a circle with a bloke in it.

So, I thought, how can this be applied to our asana while applying the rotation principle?

And this was what transpired over months of experimentation.

(My driving thought was that initially, I would only turn to the left.)

I began with Dandasana (Staff pose).

Then I crossed the right leg over the left and turned to the left, placing the left hand behind me and the right arm to the inside of the right leg, Hey presto, Ardha Matsyandrasana (Sage pose).

Now I just kept on turning. I took the weight into the right foot and placed both hands behind me then kind of moved the left foot alongside the right foot, and I had ended up facing the other end of the mat on hands and feet. Hey presto, Adho Mukha Svanasana (Dog Face Down).

Next, I stepped the right leg forward, between the hands, bent the knee and brought my abdomen to the thigh. I straightened the front leg to my own measure. Hey presto, Parsvottanasan (Intense Side Stretch).

Then I allowed the left foot to turn in a bit (to your measure or method), bent the front knee and rested the right hand inside that foot. I placed the other hand on the ear, then drove the left hand past the ear. I turned the gaze to look at the fingertips (if that's good for your neck). Wahoo – Parsvakonasana (Extended Side Pose).

Then I straightened the front leg, opened the chest to my maximum, took the left hand straight up and looked up. It's a miracle – Trikonasana (Triangle).

Then I lowered the top arm, turned the right foot in and the left foot out so that they faced the long side of the mat. I swung the torso to the centre with both hands on the floor (remember – bend your knees if you need to). This is amazing – Prasarita Paddotanasana (Wide Leg Forward Bend).

Then I brought the right hand to the centre, directly under the downwards gaze, rotated the torso and took the left hand/arm up. Turn to look up, (if it's comfy). This is becoming ridiculous – we now have Parvritti Prasarita Paddotanasana (Revolved Wide Leg Forward Bend).

Next, I turned my right foot in strongly and turned the left foot out. I swung the torso and rotated it, bringing the right hand towards the left foot. I took the left hand/arm upwards and looked up (if comfy). Now, we have Parvritti Trikonasana (Revolved Triangle).

From here, I brought the right foot alongside the left, I bent the knees and placed the right hand to the left knee, and another pose has appeared – Parvritti Utkatasa (Revolved Chair pose).

Now, I simply undid the twist of the torso, kept the knees bent and flexed at the hips; I reached the arms up, and landed in Utkatasana (Chair pose). I am astounded – where do these postures keep coming from?

I then straightened the legs, reached up, and found myself in Urdva Hastasana (Hands Up pose).

I lowered the arms – Tadasana (Tall or Mountain pose).

As stated at the beginning of this section, it was all left, so I thought, well, I shall repeat the asana but this time to the right.

But then I thought to myself, 'As I have gone from sitting in Dandasana to standing in Tadasana, why not reverse it and go from standing to sitting?' That's what I did.

When I got to sitting again, I thought, 'Better do it to the other side.' With 13 postures in the process, if you are mad, you could do it up and down; one side up and down the other side – 52 asana.

What I particularly liked was the pace at which it could be done, and that is your choice; make it as quick or as slow as you like.

Enjoy

Well, folks, that's it. I trust it has given you food for thought, and although I would encourage you to listen to your tutor, also listen to your body, as the questions it raises are well worth asking.

If I tell you something, you will stick to it and limit your own capacity to find out for yourself. (4)

Shuntya Suzuki (Not always so)

References:

1. *Kalama Sutra, attributed to the Buddha from the Pali Canon*
2. *Gustave Moreau, 1826 to 1898*
3. *Rudyard Kipling (Just so Animal Stories) 1902*
4. *Shunryu Suzuku (Not Always So) Bravo San Francisco 2003*